GW00367512

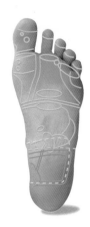

This is a Parragon Book
This edition published in 2004

PARRAGON
Queen Street House
4 Queen Street
Bath BA1 1HE, UK

Created by
THE BRIDGEWATER BOOK COMPANY

A CIP catalogue record for this book is
available from the British Library

ISBN 1-40543-926-2

Print in China

Contents

What is reflexology?

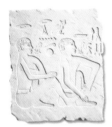

Tomb carvings suggest ancient Egyptians used reflexology.

Reflexology has been used as a holistic treatment for at least five thousand years, healing mind, body and spirit together for total health and harmony. The Chinese used pressure points on the feet as a form of treatment, and drawings discovered in the tomb of an Egyptian physician, dating back to around 2500 BC, show practitioners massaging their patients' feet and hands in a particular way.

Reflexology is a very effective form of therapy, as it can be used to diagnose various conditions as well as correcting and preventing ill health. It works on the basis that different reflex points found in the feet and hands correspond to an area in the body, and when a reflexology practitioner massages the relevant reflexes, applying pressure with the thumb and fingers in a special technique, pain and other symptoms in the corresponding area of the body are alleviated. The treatment is completely natural, and no medication is used.

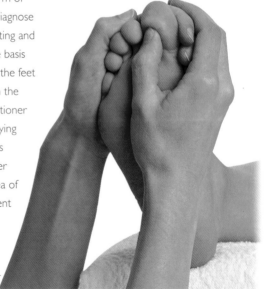

By applying pressure to specific 'reflex areas' a therapist can treat all parts of the body.

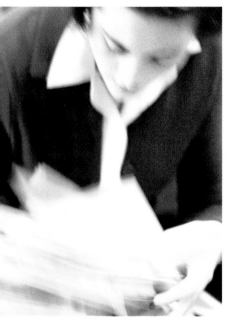

Reflexology can help to alleviate the stresses of modern living, leaving you more relaxed.

How reflexology can help you

Many physical disorders and diseases are a result of stress and lifestyle factors. People react to stress in different ways – one person may exhibit backaches, another cardiovascular problems, while another may simply become more nervous. But, whatever symptoms are experienced, everyone can benefit from reflexology.

Reflexology helps to normalise bodily functions – stimulating the elimination of waste materials from the body and improving blood circulation – and this helps to speed up the healing process. In conjunction with a reflexology treatment, a foot roller can be used to improve circulation and general well-being.

If you think reflexology may not be for you because you have ticklish or sensitive feet, don't worry – the pressure used by the practitioner is sufficiently firm for the treatment not to be ticklish, and although slight pain may be felt on some reflexes at first, the treatment as a whole will be a relaxing and enjoyable form of therapy.

People of all ages, from the very young to the elderly, can enjoy the benefits of reflexology.

How does reflexology work?

In natural medicine, the energy within us is known as the life force or vital energy. The body has ten zones – five zones on either side of the median or central line of the body. These zones are like longitudinal sections through the body, extending from front to back and containing the internal organs and glands of that section. Our vital energy is believed to flow through these zones, or energy channels, and stress, disease and injury can all lead to congestion along the energy pathways.

Every part of the foot or hand contains reflex areas, which correspond to a part of the body. If an organ is present in one or more zones, the corresponding reflex area is to be found within the same zone(s) in the hands or feet. The feet are more commonly used in reflexology as their reflexes are more responsive.

Many of the reflexes for the various organs are found on the soles of the feet and palms of the hands.

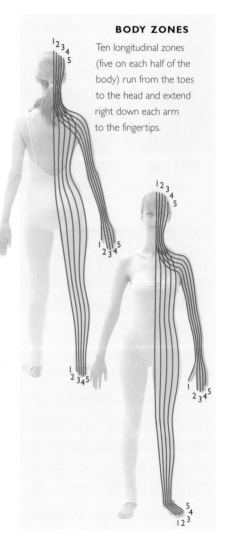

BODY ZONES

Ten longitudinal zones (five on each half of the body) run from the toes to the head and extend right down each arm to the fingertips.

FEET AND HAND ZONES

The ten zones are also found in the hands and feet, with five zones being represented on the right and five on the left.

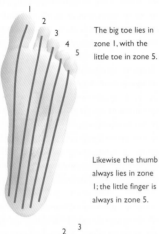

The big toe lies in zone 1, with the little toe in zone 5.

Likewise the thumb always lies in zone 1; the little finger is always in zone 5.

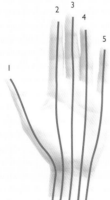

Reflexology, being a holistic therapy, uses the principle of the whole being present in each part. No one body part works in isolation, and every part of the body works together for the benefit of all. Thus the build-up of toxins in one part of the body eventually leads to different parts having to work harder to compensate for the imbalance in body energies. By stimulating the various reflexes on the feet and hands, it is possible to clear away the congestion of toxic deposits that inhibit the flow of the vital force through our bodies, bringing about a state of balance within the body and improving our health.

Exactly how massaging a reflex in the foot or hand can produce an effect on another part of the body within that zone is not fully understood, but it is accepted that a reflexology treatment has a beneficial effect on the circulation and nervous system.

Stimulating the reflexes brings improved health and vitality.

REFLEXOLOGY AND THE CIRCULATORY SYSTEM

Organs and glands that do not receive a sufficiently rich supply of blood start to malfunction, and lose their balancing qualities. The body then slowly stops being a harmonious unit.

Stress and tension have the effect of restricting blood flow. This can cause either high or low blood pressure.

Reflexology causes the body to become more relaxed. This facilitates the process of a sufficiently rich supply of blood going to the organs and glands, so that they start functioning in a more harmonious way.

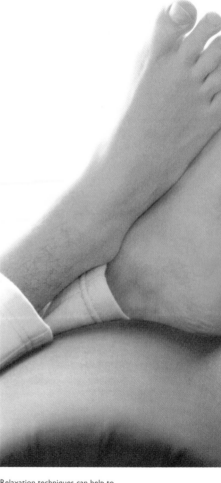

Relaxation techniques can help to ease energy blocks in the body.

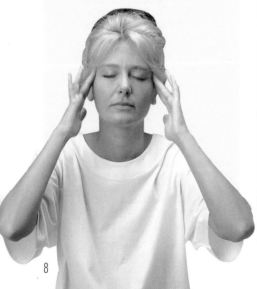

REFLEXOLOGY AND THE NERVOUS SYSTEM

The nerves, which are cord-like structures, convey impulses from the central nervous system to other parts of the body. By this type of communication they are able to co-ordinate the function of the organs and the various body parts, to work in equilibrium with one another.

Tension can put pressure on various nerves, causing messages to the organ(s) to be impaired. This has the effect of the organ not functioning as it should. Many of us have had personal experience of this, such as headaches.

Reflexology stimulates thousands of nerve endings, and thereby encourages the opening and clearing of neural pathways. Reflexology also reduces tension, and so aids the nervous system.

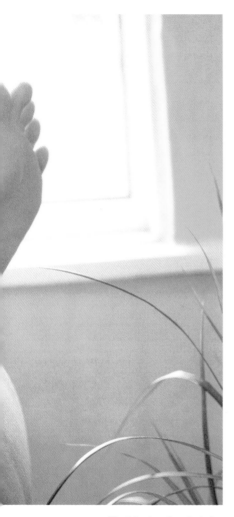

BRAIN

PERIPHERAL NERVES

Stimulating the reflexes in the feet helps to maintain optimum health.

9

Who can benefit from reflexology, and why?

A large proportion (approximately 75%) of disorders and diseases are brought about as a result of external influences, including work and lifestyle factors. People react to these stresses in various ways. For instance, one person may suffer from cardiovascular problems, while another has headaches and a third becomes anxious. Anyone who is willing to accept responsibility for their own well-being can benefit from a reflexology treatment. Reflexology does not discriminate – anyone, from youth to old age, can benefit from it.

Those with a history of cardiovascular problems should consult a doctor before having reflexology.

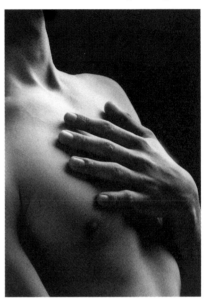

By stimulating the elimination of waste materials from the body, by improving the blood circulation or the excretory process, it is possible to speed up the healing process, thereby normalising bodily functions.

The stresses of day-to-day life can disrupt our free-flowing energy and lead to a general lack of well-being.

PRECAUTIONS

Although most disorders will benefit from a reflexology treatment, there are some conditions where reflexology is deemed to be unsuitable. These conditions include the following:

• Conditions requiring surgery

• Lymphatic cancer

• Early pregnancy (under 16 weeks), or pregnancies where there is a history of miscarriages

• More serious circulatory problems, such as phlebitis

• Deep-vein thrombosis

• Serious cases of fungal or viral foot infections, such as athlete's foot (in these instances, you could consider the option of a reflexology treatment performed on the hands)

The following conditions can be treated, but great care should be taken. If you are unsure about having reflexology alongside either of the following disorders, then you are advised not to do so.

• Heart conditions

• Epilepsy

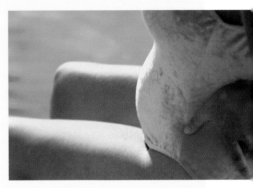

Pregnant women should generally not be given reflexology treatment.

SAFE PRACTICE

While it is safe to practise on simple problems, you are advised not to offer professional healing without training and insurance.

If you feel you have healing gifts, there are a number of schools where these gifts can be developed and guided and you can become formally qualified in the practice of reflexology.

A list of useful addresses, including relevant schools and associations of reflexology, is to be found on pages 60–61.

Reflexology is holistic
and treats each patient
as an individual.

Before you have a reflexology treatment

As reflexology is a holistic
treatment, it is important
that the therapist giving a
reflexology session treats the
person as a whole. Remember,
however, that, unless they
are licensed physicians,
reflexologists do not practise
medicine. They should never
diagnose a disease, or
prescribe or adjust any
medication you are on.
Your case history should
always be taken. Therapists
generally take some time
over this, as it not only
gives them valuable
information, but also
allows you to relax in

their company and to find out a little bit
more about reflexology.

A reflexology treatment should always
be enjoyable and relaxing, so before he or
she starts, the therapist should take time to
ensure that the environment is right.

Your lower legs should be supported,
with your feet raised and resting in
a comfortable position.

Shoes and socks should be removed.
Tight-fitting garments should be loosened
in order to allow the energy to flow
through your body.

The recipient normally
sits in a reclining chair,
with the feet at a height
that is convenient for
the therapist.

The session can now begin

Everyone's feet are different, and the therapist can gain much information from the general appearance, colour and temperature of your feet. Cold feet that are rather blue or red indicate poor circulation. Feet that perspire indicate a glandular imbalance. Dry skin on the feet again indicates poor circulation. Cracks in

Foot problems, such as fungal conditions, should be treated before having reflexology.

the soles, calluses, corns and bunions should be noted, and the area where they occur; for example, cracks on the heel indicate pelvic disorders. And the therapist should look at the zones on the feet in which these problems occur, as they will be linked to the body zone of the same number. An ingrowing toenail may relate to headaches or migraine. Flat feet may indicate a problem with the spine. Varicose veins should not be worked on directly, as it is possible that further damage could occur. The therapist should check to make sure that you do not suffer from extensive fungal infection, as this could easily pass to their hands. They should not work where verrucas exist, as these can rapidly spread to other areas of the foot, or may be passed on to them.

Reactions to reflexology

Once the treatment has finished, you should feel relaxed and often warmer, owing to the stimulation of the blood circulation. Sometimes, however, you may feel cold – this is because of the toxins leaving your body.

In order for the body to heal itself, it has to get rid of toxic substances. The degree of healing crisis depends upon the person and their imbalances. So that you do not have too strong a healing crisis, it is always best if the therapist gives a gentle first treatment, and observes you and

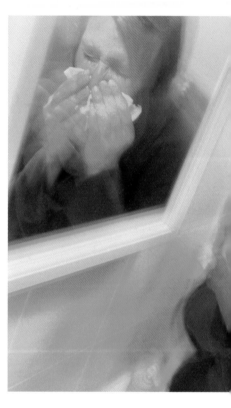

Individuals react in different ways after treatment. Minor side-effects include feeling cold and slight nausea.

your reactions before the second treatment is given, which can then be tailor-made to your needs.

Most forms of disease have been building up over a period of time. It is, therefore, unrealistic to expect an instantaneous improvement.

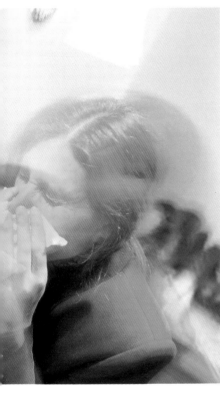

Some patients have a runny nose after treatment, as a result of the sinuses clearing and expelling mucus.

Here are some of the more common reactions that may occur:
• Perhaps the most usual one is that you have a very good night's sleep.
• Your rate of urination may increase. The colour and smell may also change.
• You may get a cold.
• Some people experience a headache. If this does occur, it is best not to take any medication to suppress it.
• Suppressed medical conditions could flare up again.

These are all positive reactions, and show that your body is trying to heal itself. The healing crisis is usually short-lived, leaving you with a heightened feeling of well-being.

Some people may feel tired for a day or so after treatment.

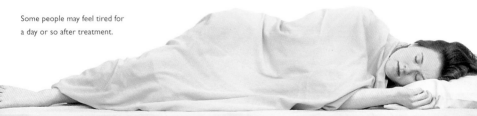

NUMBER OF TREATMENTS REQUIRED

Every person is different, so it is not possible to predict the exact number of sessions that will be required. For all diseases, an entire course of reflexology treatment is recommended, even if the symptoms appear to go after the first treatment. The course of treatment will help to balance the body's systems, which will in turn help to prevent a recurrence of the disorder.

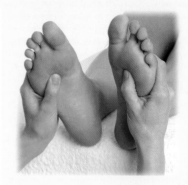

Usually some sort of improvement should occur after about three sessions. If after four sessions there does not seem to be any noticeable change, then perhaps reflexology is not going to be of help in your particular case. However, there are very few people who have experienced a reflexology treatment that has been properly administered and who have not benefited in some way.

Enjoy the process of receiving your reflexology treatment. It will be a marvellous hour of health-giving and relaxation for you.

The whole body should be feeling relaxed and more flexible at the end of a treatment session.

USING REFLEXOLOGY ROLLERS

Massaging your soles and palms with a reflexology roller will:

- relieve aches and pains
- invigorate tired feet and hands
- prepare feet and hands for reflexology treatment.

Make sure your feet and hands are clean before massaging. In fact, this self-treatment is ideal following a bath or shower.

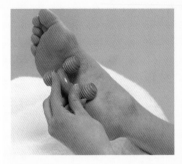

USING A CYLINDRICAL ROLLER

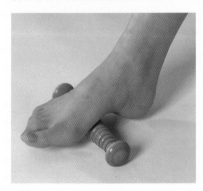

STEP 1 Sit comfortably with both feet flat on the floor, about a shoulder-width apart.

STEP 2 Place the roller horizontally under your right foot and roll your foot over it, from toes to heel and back again, for as long as it feels comfortable.

STEP 3 Repeat with your left foot.

USING A HAND-HELD ROLLER

STEP 1 Sit comfortably with your right foot resting on the knee of your left leg.

STEP 2 Move the roller up and down the sole of your right foot, applying as much pressure as you feel comfortable with, particularly to the ball and heel.

STEP 3 Repeat on your left foot.

STEP 4 Rub the roller up and down your right palm, applying particularly firm pressure to the heel (the fleshy area below the thumb).

STEP 5 Repeat on your left palm.

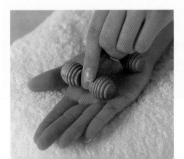

Anatomy

All the body's systems need to work together harmoniously to produce a healthy person. Diet and exercise are also essential for optimum health.

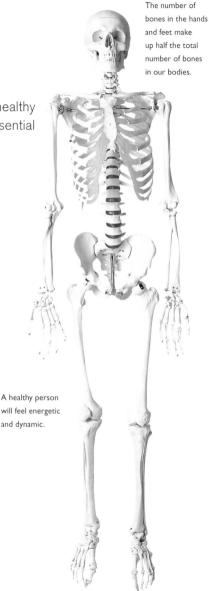

The number of bones in the hands and feet make up half the total number of bones in our bodies.

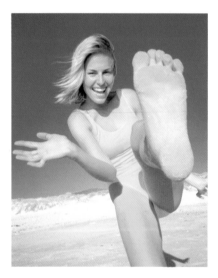

A healthy person will feel energetic and dynamic.

Skeletal system

The bones give the body support and protect the internal glands and organs. They give the body shape and regulate the body's minerals. In the bone marrow, red and white blood cells as well as platelets are manufactured.

Nervous system

The nervous system is made up of two parts:

• The central nervous system. This consists of the brain and spinal cord.

• The peripheral nervous system. This carries information from various parts of the body to the central nervous system through the afferent sensory nerves, and carries out instructions through the efferent motor nerves. The nerves are made up of thousands of long, thin nerve fibres.

BRAIN

SPINAL CORD

PERIPHERAL NERVES

The brain controls the complex nervous system of the body.

Muscular system

Muscles are composed of tissue, which can be contracted so that movement can occur. They make up between 35 and 45% of body weight. There are three types of muscle tissue:

• Skeletal muscle. This is under the conscious control of the person concerned. There are more than 650 skeletal muscles in the body.

• Cardiac muscle. This type is only found in the heart.

• Smooth muscle. This is found in the intestines.

FLEXORS OF THE WRIST AND FINGERS

QUADRICEPS FEMORIS MUSCLE STRAIGHTENS THE KNEE

The body contains an intricate network of muscles, which work in association with each other.

Circulatory system

The heart, an organ about the size of a clenched fist, is situated in the thorax. The heart pumps deoxygenated blood to the lungs; here carbon dioxide and oxygen are exchanged. This happens through the alveolar surface (a thin-walled air-filled sac that is surrounded by blood capillaries) of the lung. Oxygenated blood returns to the heart. This is known as the pulmonary circulation. The systemic circulation carries the oxygenated blood and nutrition to all the other parts of the body, returning with the waste products that have to be filtered and excreted. Carbon dioxide is also returned to the heart by the systemic circulatory system, where, after being pumped through the heart chambers, it enters the pulmonary circulatory system, and so the process starts again.

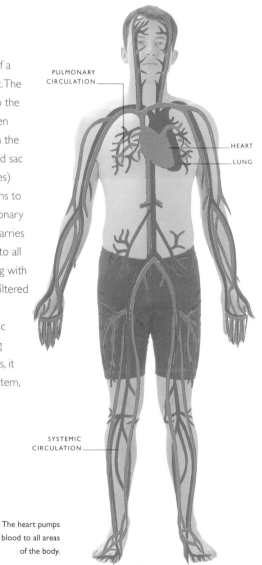

PULMONARY
CIRCULATION

HEART

LUNG

SYSTEMIC
CIRCULATION

The heart pumps
blood to all areas
of the body.

Respiratory system

The human respiratory system is made up of the nose and mouth, the pharynx and larynx in the throat, and the windpipe or trachea. The trachea then divides into two bronchi, which enter the lungs. The bronchi subdivide into smaller bronchioles, and they in turn subdivide into the alveolar ducts of the alveolar sacs, which contain the individual alveoli. The main muscles used in breathing are the intercostal muscles; these run in between the ribs and the diaphragm.

Respiration in humans is the process whereby oxygen is used during metabolism to produce carbon dioxide. This gaseous exchange occurs through the alveoli in the lungs.

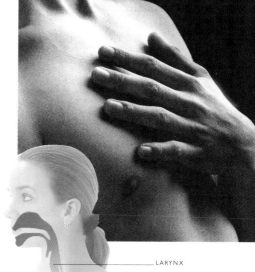

LARYNX

TRACHEA

LUNG

DIAPHRAGM

A healthy respiratory system helps to promote a general sense of well-being.

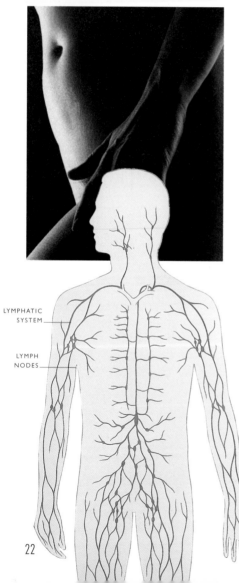

LYMPHATIC
SYSTEM

LYMPH
NODES

Lymphatic system

This is our defence system for protecting the body from bacteria and other organisms. Lymph is transported by the lymphatic system, and lymph nodes are situated at intervals along the lymphatics. The lymph nodes contain a system of narrow channels through which the lymph drains. Along the walls of these channels large phagocytes (these are cells that engulf particles) surround bacteria, other harmful substances and dead cells from the lymph. Large lymph nodes are found in the neck, under the arms, in the breast and in the groin. The large lymphatics unite into two lymphatic ducts, which then drain into the bloodstream. The spleen and the thymus are also part of the lymphatic system. The spleen is a large, vascular, ductless organ found on the left side of the body behind the stomach. It plays an important part in the immune system, producing lymphocytes (white blood cells), and is involved in the breakdown and recycling of haemoglobin from old blood cells.

Lymph vessels are a vital component of the body's immune system.

Endocrine system

The endocrine system consists of ductless glands, which produce and secrete hormones directly into the bloodstream. These hormones are carried in the blood until they affect those organs that are sensitive to them. Both the nervous system and the endocrine system co-ordinate the body's activities, but they do this in different ways.

The endocrine glands include the pituitary gland, which is found in the brain. The activity of the pituitary is regulated by the hypothalamus. The pituitary gland controls the function of the thyroid, adrenals and the reproductive glands (consisting of the ovaries and testes).

The parathyroid glands, pancreas, placenta and gastrointestinal mucosa are also part of the endocrine system.

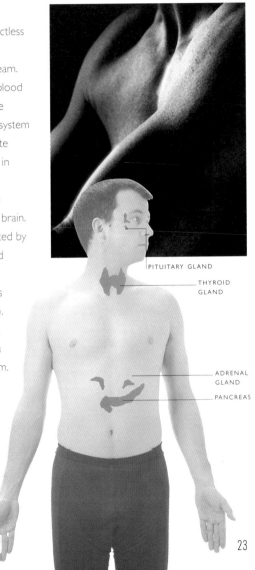

PITUITARY GLAND

THYROID GLAND

ADRENAL GLAND

PANCREAS

The endocrine system controls the body's secretion of hormones.

Urinary system

The urinary system consists of two kidneys, situated one on either side of the spine. They filter the blood, and regulate the composition and volume of the body fluids by eliminating what cannot be reused, such as salts, waste products and excess water. Renal arteries and veins bring a rich blood supply to and from the kidneys. The kidneys are connected to the bladder by the ureter tubes. Urine continuously drains out of the kidneys into the ureters and into the bladder. The constant flow of urine into the bladder causes it to swell. The bladder wall contains sensory nerve endings, which send messages to the brain, alerting you when the bladder needs emptying. By relaxing the sphincter muscle around the urethra, urination can then occur.

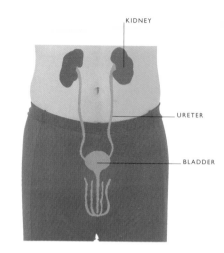

Some men have difficulty emptying the bladder as a result of an enlarged prostate.

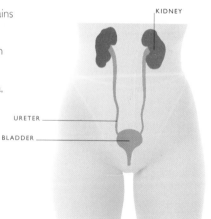

Cystitis (bladder infection) is more common in women.

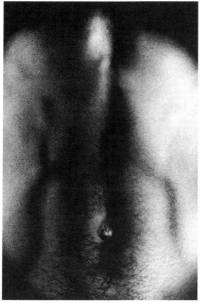

more absorbable state. The mixture then enters the small intestine, followed by the large intestine, where further breakdown and absorption take place. The unabsorbed residue is finally expelled through the rectum and anus.

The liver, gall bladder and pancreas are also important in the digestion process.

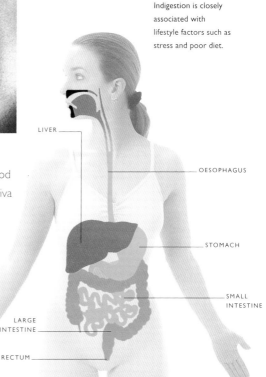

Indigestion is closely associated with lifestyle factors such as stress and poor diet.

LIVER

OESOPHAGUS

STOMACH

SMALL INTESTINE

LARGE INTESTINE

RECTUM

Digestive system

Digestion starts in the mouth, where food is chewed and mixed with saliva. The saliva lubricates the food, making it softer and easier to swallow.

The ingested food then enters the oesophagus and goes to the stomach. Here it is churned and mixed with the stomach acids to change the food substances into a

Reproductive system

The majority of the male reproductive anatomy is external. The two testes hang in scrotal sacs. Two long convoluted tubes, one on each side, called the epididymis, are attached to the testes. These allow the sperm, which have been produced in the testes, to ripen. The epididymis then opens into the vas deferens, again two long tubes, one on each side of the body, which are joined to the seminal vesicles. The seminal vesicles act as a storage place for mature sperm before being released through the centre of the prostate gland and to the exterior by the urethra.

The female reproductive organs consist of the ovaries, Fallopian tubes, the uterus and the breasts.

The testes and ovaries produce reproductive cells called, respectively, spermatozoa and ova. They also produce the hormones that influence body development and behaviour.

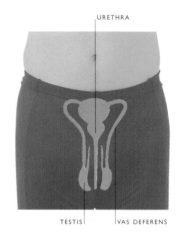

URETHRA

TESTIS | VAS DEFERENS

Reflexology can help to alleviate prostate problems in men.

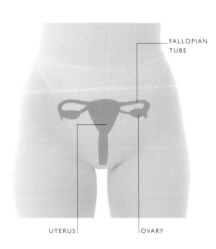

FALLOPIAN TUBE

UTERUS | OVARY

Menstrual difficulties can be alleviated by using reflexology in the wrist and ankle areas.

Sensory system

The sense organs allow the body to be aware of its environment by working in the following way. When a sensory cell is stimulated, electrical impulses are sent by means of nerves to the brain. Once they arrive at the appropriate part of the brain they are interpreted as sight, sound, pain, and so on. The skin, the eyes, the ears, the nose and the tongue are all part of the sensory system.

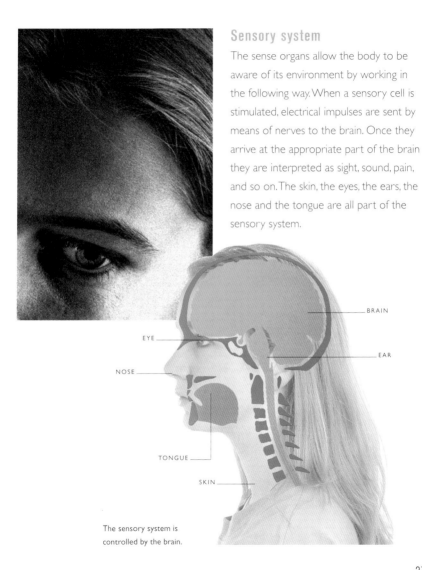

BRAIN

EYE

EAR

NOSE

TONGUE

SKIN

The sensory system is controlled by the brain.

Reflex mapping

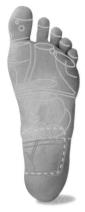

One of the most important steps of reflexology is a thorough understanding of the feet in relation to the body. The feet are like a mini-map of the whole body. All the organs, glands and various body parts are imaged on the feet in almost the same arrangement as in the body. Reflex areas are found on the soles, sides and tops of the feet. The hands also contain reflex areas on their palms, sides and backs.

Reflexologists map the different zones of the feet.

The body is divided into two halves. The right foot represents the right side of the body, with the medial (inside) of the foot representing the right half of the spine. The left foot represents the left side of the body, again with the medial representing the left half of the spine.

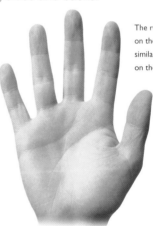

The reflex areas on the hands are similar to those on the feet.

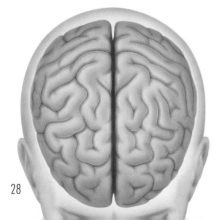

Perhaps it should be pointed out that the right side of the brain is located on the right foot and the left side on the left foot. The zones do not cross in the brain, as the nervous system does.

The brain has two hemispheres controlling different body functions.

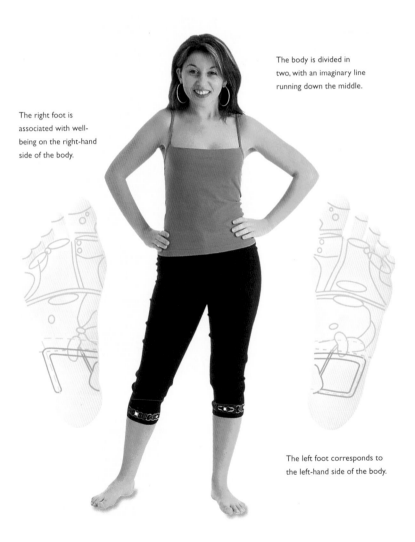

The body is divided in
two, with an imaginary line
running down the middle.

The right foot is
associated with well-
being on the right-hand
side of the body.

The left foot corresponds to
the left-hand side of the body.

29

The eight sections of the foot

Each foot is divided into five longitudinal zones, with each zone containing a toe. The foot is then further subdivided into eight sections.

• The head and neck are represented by the toes. The right foot represents the right side of the head with its associated organs, and the left foot represents the left side of the head with its various organs.

• The thoracic and upper abdominal area is represented by the area between the base of the toes and the base of the metatarsal bones (waistline). This can be more easily located by running a horizontal line across the foot from the bony protrusion on the side of the foot (cuboid notch).

• The lower abdominal area, stretching from the lower part of the stomach and kidneys to the pelvic area, is represented on the foot by the area between the waistline and the pelvic line. This is located by connecting the inner and outer ankle bone protrusions (which are known as the malleoli), going under the foot. So the reflexes of the abdomen and pelvis are found over the tarsal bones and around the ankle bones.

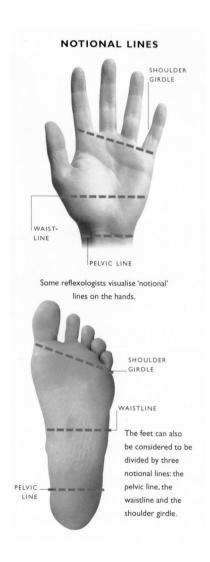

NOTIONAL LINES

SHOULDER GIRDLE

WAIST-LINE

PELVIC LINE

Some reflexologists visualise 'notional' lines on the hands.

SHOULDER GIRDLE

WAISTLINE

PELVIC LINE

The feet can also be considered to be divided by three notional lines: the pelvic line, the waistline and the shoulder girdle.

• The pelvic area is represented by the heel, starting from the pelvic line and running to the rear of the heel.

• The reproductive area is represented by parts of the ankle.

• The spine is represented by the instep. The spine's curve closely resembles the natural sweep of the instep.

• The limbs are represented by the outer edges of the foot.

• The reflexes for the breast and lymphatic system are on the top of the foot.

We can now look more closely at the arrangement of reflexes in the feet. All the reflexes on the following pages are found on both feet, unless otherwise stated.

HORIZONTAL ZONES

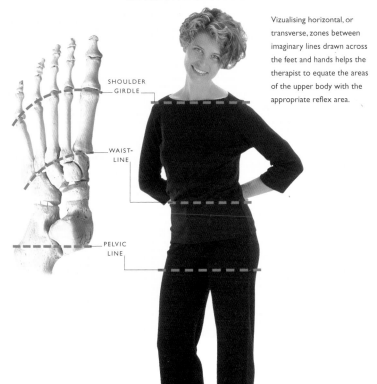

SHOULDER GIRDLE

WAIST-LINE

PELVIC LINE

Vizualising horizontal, or transverse, zones between imaginary lines drawn across the feet and hands helps the therapist to equate the areas of the upper body with the appropriate reflex area.

The head

The brain is represented by the tip of the big toes. Areas on the other toes aid in fine-tuning reflexology treatment to the head. Babies, children and the elderly all react well to light pressure on these reflexes.

The pituitary gland reflex is found approximately in the middle of the fleshy part of the big toe of both feet, at the centre of the toe-print whorl.

• The reflexes for the sinuses are found in the other four toes.

• The eye reflex is located at the base of the second and third toes, just below the point where the toes join the ball of the foot.

• The ear reflex is found at the base of the fourth and fifth toes, just below where the toes join the ball of the foot.

• The Eustachian tube reflex is found just below the web, between the third and fourth toes.

• The face is represented by the front of the big toe.

• The teeth and gum reflexes are found on the front of the four small toes, with different teeth being represented by different toes.

• The neck reflex is found between the fleshy part of the big toe and the fleshy pad of the ball of the foot.

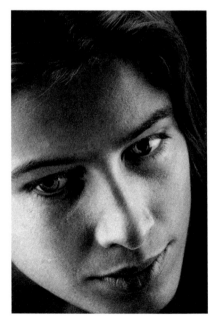

Facial, eye, ear and teeth problems are treated using reflexes on the toes.

HEAD REFLEXES

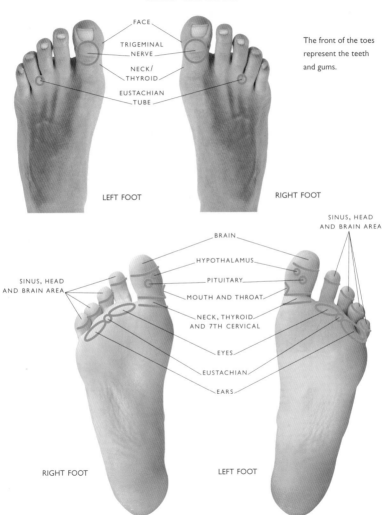

FACE

TRIGEMINAL
NERVE

NECK/
THYROID

EUSTACHIAN
TUBE

LEFT FOOT

RIGHT FOOT

The front of the toes
represent the teeth
and gums.

SINUS, HEAD
AND BRAIN AREA

BRAIN

HYPOTHALAMUS

PITUITARY

MOUTH AND THROAT

NECK, THYROID
AND 7TH CERVICAL

EYES

EUSTACHIAN

EARS

SINUS, HEAD
AND BRAIN AREA

RIGHT FOOT

LEFT FOOT

33

The thoracic and upper abdominal area

This area covers the entire region of the body from the shoulder girdle down to the kidneys. As such, it incorporates several vital reflexes, such as those of the lung, heart and liver.

The shoulder reflex is found around the base of the little toe, on the sole, outer side and top of the foot. It extends from the base of the toes to about halfway down the fifth metatarsal.

• The lung reflex is found across zones 2 to 5, over the metatarsal bones of the foot. Both the sole and the top of the foot act as a reflex for the lung. Reflexes for the trachea and bronchi, as well as the oesophagus, are found in a roughly vertical line between the big toes and second toes.

• The diaphragm reflex is found on the soles, following a line along the ball of the foot, halfway up the metatarsal bones, across all five zones.

• The heart reflex is located in the left foot only, in zones 2 and 3, just above the diaphragm reflex.

• The thyroid reflex is found in zone 1 on the upper part of the ball of the foot.

• The parathyroid reflexes are closely linked with the thyroid reflexes. An upper and lower parathyroid reflex is found in both feet.

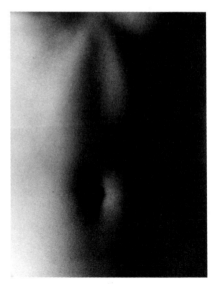

The reflex for the diaphragm is found on the soles of the feet.

THORACIC AND UPPER ABDOMINAL REFLEXES

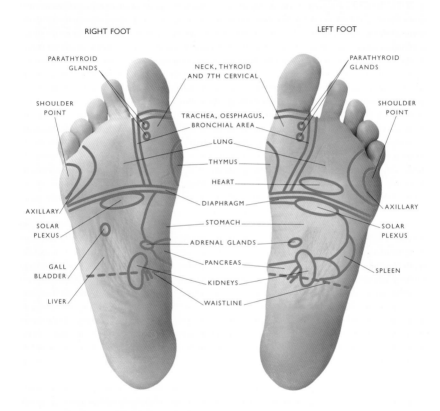

RIGHT FOOT

LEFT FOOT

PARATHYROID
GLANDS

NECK, THYROID
AND 7TH CERVICAL

PARATHYROID
GLANDS

SHOULDER
POINT

TRACHEA, OESPHAGUS,
BRONCHIAL AREA

SHOULDER
POINT

LUNG

THYMUS

HEART

DIAPHRAGM

AXILLARY

AXILLARY

SOLAR
PLEXUS

STOMACH

SOLAR
PLEXUS

ADRENAL GLANDS

GALL
BLADDER

PANCREAS

SPLEEN

KIDNEYS

LIVER

WAISTLINE

The reflexes for the thoracic and upper abdominal area are
spread over much of the soles of the feet.

• The thymus gland reflex is found in zone
I on both feet, over the ball of the big toe.
• The solar plexus reflex is found at the
same level as the diaphragm in zones
2–3. This reflex is used to induce a relaxed
state. It can relieve stress and nervousness.
• The liver reflex is found on the sole of
the right foot, between the diaphragm
reflex and the waistline, where it fills most
of this area.
• The gall bladder reflex is found in zone
4 on the right foot, in the liver area.
• The stomach reflex is located on the
soles of both feet. On the left foot, the reflex
occupies zones I to 4; on the right foot it
occupies zones I to 2. The stomach is
found between the diaphragm and waistline.
• The pancreas reflex is similar to the
stomach reflex, being located in zones
I to 4 on the left foot and in zones
I to 2 on the right foot. It is found from
the waistline to about halfway up towards
the diaphragm.
• The spleen reflex is found on the left
foot between zones 4 and 5 at a similar
horizontal level to the stomach.
• The kidney reflexes are found on the
soles of both feet, at about waistline level
in zones 2 to 3. The right kidney is slightly
lower than the left kidney, both in the body
itself and in the positioning of its reflexes.
• The adrenal gland reflexes are found on
the soles of both feet, just above and
slightly to the inside of the kidney reflex
in zone I.

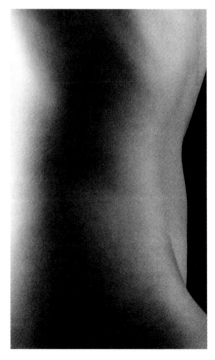

Stomach complaints are a good
candidate for reflexology treatment.

THORACIC AND UPPER ABDOMINAL REFLEXES

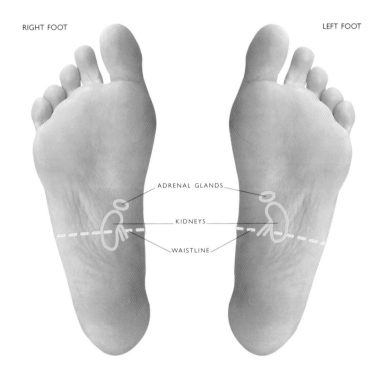

RIGHT FOOT

LEFT FOOT

ADRENAL GLANDS

KIDNEYS

WAISTLINE

The kidney and adrenal gland reflexes are positioned very
specifically on and just above the waistline.

The lower abdominal area

This area includes the reflexes for the bladder and ureter, as well as the complex reflex for the large intestine. If this body organ is not functioning properly, diarrhoea and constipation may result.

The small intestine reflex is found on the soles of both feet, in between the waistline and pelvic line from zones 1 to 4.

• The ileo-caecal valve reflex is found on the right sole, in the line between zones 4 and 5, just above the pelvic line.

• The appendix reflex is found at the same location as the ileo-caecal valve.

• The large intestine reflexes are found on both feet. On the right foot this begins just below the reflex for the appendix and ileo-caecal valve. It extends upwards (representing the ascending colon), turning just below the waistline to become the transverse colon, which goes across the entire foot, extending to the left foot; it then turns at the end of zone 5 to become the descending colon. Just above the pelvic line another turn is made into the sigmoid colon; this drops down to the pelvic line at zone 3, ending at the rectum reflex.

• The ureter reflex is found on the soles of both feet. As expected, it links the kidney reflexes to the bladder reflex. This reflex passes from zones 2 to 1.

• The bladder reflex is found on the soles of both feet. It is often seen as a puffy area in zone 1 on the inner side of the foot.

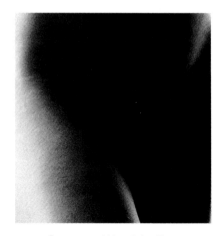

For someone with intestinal problems the right foot is usually treated first.

LOWER ABDOMINAL REFLEXES

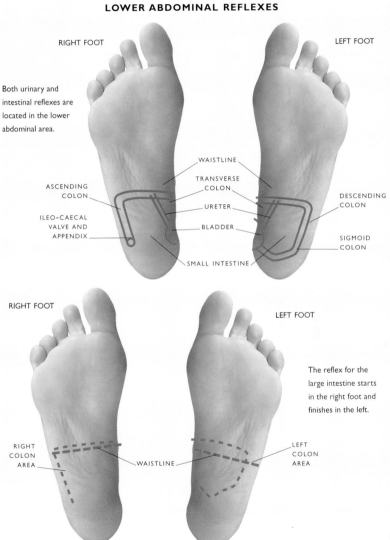

RIGHT FOOT

LEFT FOOT

Both urinary and intestinal reflexes are located in the lower abdominal area.

WAISTLINE

TRANSVERSE COLON

ASCENDING COLON

URETER

DESCENDING COLON

ILEO-CAECAL VALVE AND APPENDIX

BLADDER

SIGMOID COLON

SMALL INTESTINE

RIGHT FOOT

LEFT FOOT

The reflex for the large intestine starts in the right foot and finishes in the left.

RIGHT COLON AREA

WAISTLINE

LEFT COLON AREA

39

The pelvic area

This region is significant because the largest nerve in the body, the sciatic nerve, starts here, running down the buttocks and thighs to supply the lower legs and feet.

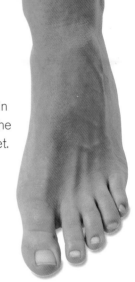

The sciatic nerve reflex is found along the sciatic nerve itself, across the heel, about one-third of the way down. It is located on the soles of both feet, and a few centimetres up the ankle on either side of the Achilles tendon.

PELVIC REFLEXES

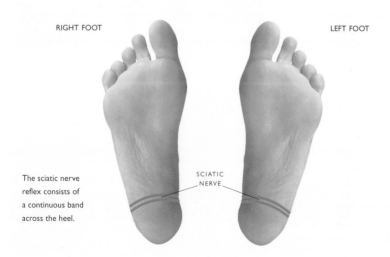

RIGHT FOOT

LEFT FOOT

The sciatic nerve reflex consists of a continuous band across the heel.

SCIATIC NERVE

The reproductive area

It should be noted that the reflexes for the ovaries in women are at the same position as those for the testes in men. Likewise, the position of the uterus reflex in women corresponds to the prostate gland in men.

The ovary/testes reflexes are found on the outer side of both feet, halfway between the ankle bone and the back of the heel. The heel itself is a helper area.

• The uterus and prostate reflexes are found midway between the ankle bone and heel, on the inner side of each foot.

• The Fallopian tube and seminal vesicle/vas deferens reflexes again occupy the same area in males and females. They are found across the top of the foot, linking one ankle bone to the other.

REPRODUCTIVE REFLEXES

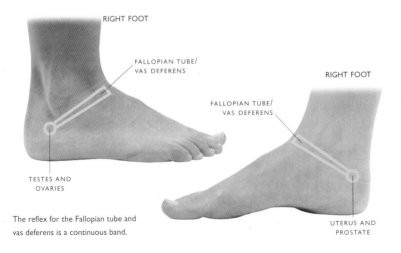

RIGHT FOOT

FALLOPIAN TUBE/
VAS DEFERENS

RIGHT FOOT

FALLOPIAN TUBE/
VAS DEFERENS

TESTES AND
OVARIES

UTERUS AND
PROSTATE

The reflex for the Fallopian tube and vas deferens is a continuous band.

The spine

The spine, enclosing the spinal cord, comprises five sections — the cervical vertebrae, thoracic vertebrae, lumbar vertebrae, sacrum and coccyx. They are represented on the foot by five areas on the spine reflex.

The spine reflexes are found down the inner sides of both feet. The cervical area lies between the top of the side of the big toe and the base of the big toe. The side of the first metatarsal bone represents the thoracic vertebrae, with the lumbar vertebrae reflex being found from the waistline of the foot to about the inner ankle bone.

• The rest of the inner side of the foot corresponds to the sacrum and coccyx at the base of the spine.

SPINE REFLEXES

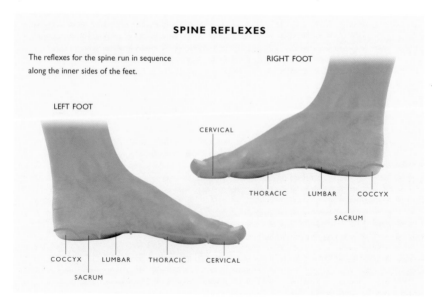

The reflexes for the spine run in sequence along the inner sides of the feet.

RIGHT FOOT

LEFT FOOT

CERVICAL

THORACIC   LUMBAR   COCCYX

SACRUM

COCCYX   LUMBAR   THORACIC   CERVICAL

SACRUM

Other areas

Reflexes situated on the outside and top of the foot correspond to outer parts of the body, such as the elbow and knee, as well as to the breasts and the lymph nodes.

The outer foot

• The upper arm reflex can be found on the outer side of the foot, under the shoulder reflex and the cuboid notch.
• The elbow reflex is represented by the cuboid notch.
• The pelvic reflex is found over the tarsal bones of both feet.
• The knee reflex is found below the pelvis reflex on the outer side of the foot.

The top of the foot

• The breast reflex is situated at the top of the foot, behind the toes to about the waistline level.
• The upper lymph node reflexes are found in between the toes. Stimulating the lymphatic drainage system back to the venous system may be done by the therapist working on both feet, on the tops and soles between the toes, using a pinching action.

OTHER REFLEXES

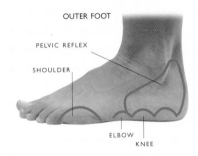

OUTER FOOT

PELVIC REFLEX

SHOULDER

ELBOW

KNEE

TOP OF FOOT

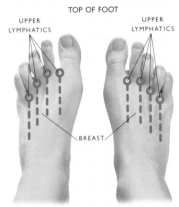

UPPER LYMPHATICS

UPPER LYMPHATICS

BREAST

43

The massage technique

Once you are familiar with the reflexes of the feet, and the areas of the body to which they correspond, you can focus on the techniques. You may wish to train in reflexology yourself. What follows will give you an insight into the treatment you receive and may one day yourself give.

After ensuring that the client is not allergic to talcum powder, apply a small amount to the feet. Oil makes the surface of the foot too slippery for reflexology. The reflexology massage technique is mainly done with the thumb; both right and left thumbs are used at different times. The fingers do, however, have a part to play at various times. The thumb is bent at an angle of about 45° and walks along the foot in very small steps, doing the caterpillar walk.

Each reflex is about the size of a pinhead so, for the treatment to be effective, precision is required. The pressure used should be firm, not agonising. The hands and fingers are also used to support the foot and sometimes to provide leverage.

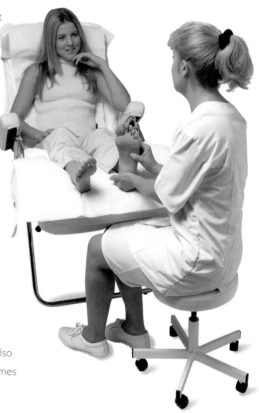

The client may feel a variety of sensations. Any tenderness felt over the congested areas will diminish with successive treatments. Although some pain may be felt on some of the reflexes, the treatment as a whole should not be painful and should leave the client feeling relaxed and refreshed.

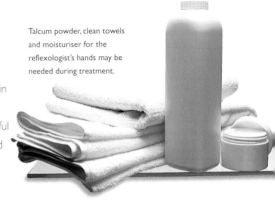

Talcum powder, clean towels and moisturiser for the reflexologist's hands may be needed during treatment.

After applying talcum powder to the feet, the left foot can be covered with a towel to keep it warm.

The relaxation technique (see pages 46–49) eases the foot before treatment. The circulation is stimulated and the technique allows the client to become accustomed to your touch. Both feet can be relaxed, then the main treatment can start on the right foot. Or the right foot can be relaxed and then worked on, followed by the left foot.

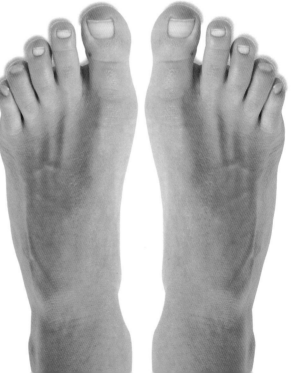

The feet should be dry and free of blisters and cuts before treatment begins.

Relaxing the foot

Various different techniques can be used to relax the foot prior to treatment. This is especially useful if the client is anxious about reflexology, or if certain areas of the body are tense and under strain.

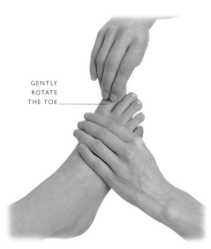

GENTLY
ROTATE
THE TOE

Metatarsal kneading

With one hand holding the foot at the toes, clench the other hand to form a fist. Starting at the fleshy part of the sole just under the toes, use your fist to push against the foot in a kneading motion. Move down the foot to the heel, moving the other hand down at the same time to maintain support of the client's foot. This kneading can be repeated a few times.

Toe rotation

Starting with the big toe, hold the toe with your finger and thumb of one hand, with the other hand supporting the foot itself. Gently rotate the toe in one direction three times, then rotate it in the opposite direction three times. Give it a gentle tug. Then repeat for the other toes, working in sequence to the little toe.

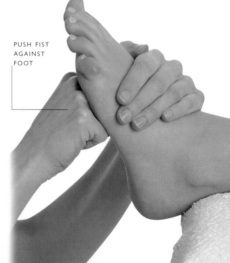

PUSH FIST
AGAINST
FOOT

PLACE ONE
THUMB ABOVE
THE OTHER

PLACE FINGERS
OVER FRONT
OF FOOT

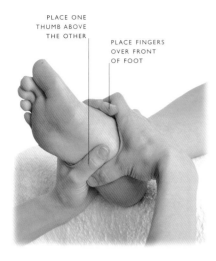

Thumb-rolling

Hold the foot by placing both sets of
fingers over the top of the foot, with the
thumbs on the sole, one above the other,
at the base of the heel. Then firmly and
smoothly place the bottom thumb above
the top one. Continue this process until
the area from the heel to the base of the
toes has been thumb-rolled.

TIP

Do not rotate the big toe too
vigorously, as it corresponds to the neck
area and could leave the client feeling
uncomfortable. Likewise, be gentle in
the way you rotate the foot during
the spinal twist.

Spinal twist

Place the fingers of both hands side by
side, holding the top of the foot by the
ankle, with the thumbs on the sole, in a
position similar to that when a 'Chinese
burn' is given to the wrist. The hand closest
to the heel is kept still, while the other
hand slowly and smoothly rotates the foot
back and forth. Ensure that the foot is
rotated evenly in both directions.

Repeat this a few times, then edge
towards the toes, using the same technique.
Continue until you reach the toes.

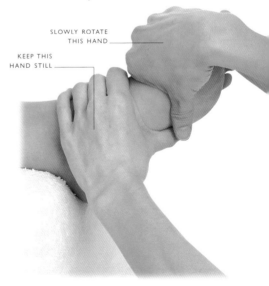

SLOWLY ROTATE
THIS HAND

KEEP THIS
HAND STILL

47

Ankle rotation

Cup the heel in one hand, and with the other hand firmly hold the toes and part of the sole. Keeping your cupped hand still, gently rotate the foot clockwise in complete circles a few times, then anti-clockwise. This action, as well as being a relaxation technique, works on the reflex of the uterus and the prostate, and the whole of the hip area.

HOLD THE
TOES FIRMLY

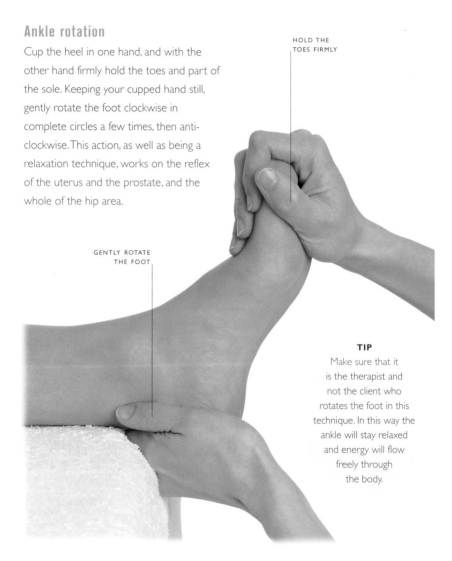

GENTLY ROTATE
THE FOOT

TIP

Make sure that it is the therapist and not the client who rotates the foot in this technique. In this way the ankle will stay relaxed and energy will flow freely through the body.

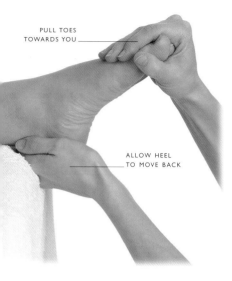

PULL TOES
TOWARDS YOU

ALLOW HEEL
TO MOVE BACK

Foot wobbling

Place one palm on each side of the ankle, at right angles to the foot. Keeping the hands and wrists relaxed, rock the foot from side to side by gently moving your hands back and forth in opposite directions. Gradually move your hands up from the ankle to the toes so that the whole of the foot is worked. This technique is good for relaxing the foot and lower leg. It also aids circulation.

Achilles' tendon stretch

Cup the heel in one hand. Grasp the top of the foot near the toes. Pull the toes towards you, allowing the heel to move backwards, then pull the heel towards you, allowing the toes to move backwards. Repeat this action a few times.

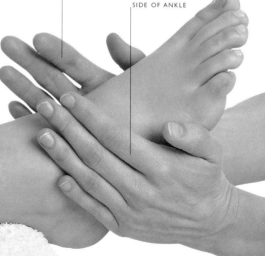

MOVE HANDS
BACK AND FORTH

PLACE PALMS
ON EITHER
SIDE OF ANKLE

49

The main treatment

This is the sequence for the main reflexology treatment. It is worth asking the client what sensations they are experiencing during treatment – these may be emotional as well as physical. When a client tells you that an area is tender, release the pressure slightly and rework the area. Do the same if you notice any blockages, which may feel like sand under the skin.

Starting with the right foot

EYE AND EAR REFLEX

1 *With the thumb in the bent position, as previously described, pinch the hypothalamus reflex by placing the hand over the toes, the fingers over the front of the big toe and the thumb over the reflex, and using a pinching-type squeezing motion. Repeat for the pituitary reflex.*

HYPOTHALAMUS REFLEX

3 *Caterpillar walk over the eye and ear reflex in both directions. Work over the Eustachian reflex, using a pinching and circular motion with the thumb and index finger.*

SIDE OF THE
HEAD REFLEX

2 *Caterpillar walk (see page 44) over the toes, starting with the sole of the big toe and walking upwards, then across the face reflex. Go up the back of the other toes and down the front, working in sequence to the little toe. Caterpillar walk over the top of the toes in both directions., and over the neck reflex.*

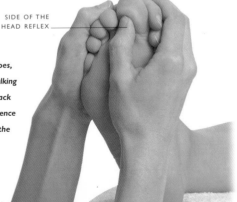

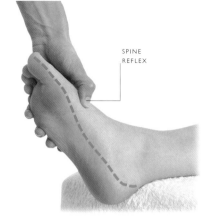

SPINE
REFLEX

6 Work the outer foot. Starting at the base of the little toe, work the arm, elbow and knee, ending with the hip reflex. Work the cuboid notch in both directions. The hip reflex should also be worked in a criss-cross manner.

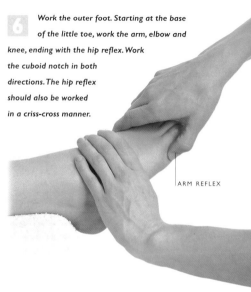

ARM REFLEX

4 Work up and down the spine reflex, using the caterpillar walk. At the heel part, slightly increase the pressure you are using. Many people find parts of this reflex tender.

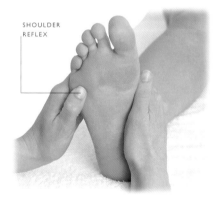

SHOULDER
REFLEX

7 Stimulate the thyroid and parathyroid by using a circular motion with the thumb.

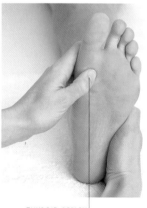

5 Work the shoulder reflex. Start low down on the sole, doing the caterpillar walk with the thumb and working towards the toes. Then do the front part of the shoulder reflex, with the index finger doing the caterpillar walk this time. The shoulder reflex often feels rather crunchy, again because of tension that is found in this area.

THYROID REFLEX

8   *Caterpillar walk over the trachea and oesophagus reflex.*

9   *Caterpillar walk the sole part of the lung reflex, while putting your left-hand thumb over the diaphragm reflex, with the fingers over the front of the foot. Work this reflex both up and down. Then caterpillar walk the front part of the foot, from zone 5 to zone 1, over the lung reflex.*

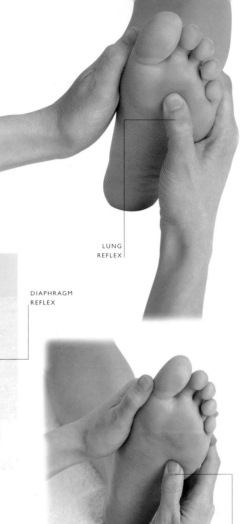

LUNG
REFLEX

DIAPHRAGM
REFLEX

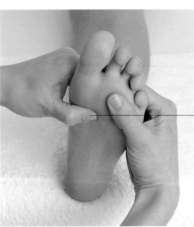

10   *Caterpillar walk over the diaphragm reflex in both directions.*

11   *Work the spleen and stomach reflex by caterpillar walking across zones 1 to 2.*

SPLEEN AND
STOMACH
REFLEX

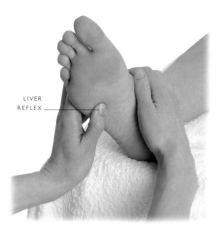

SMALL
INTESTINE
REFLEX

LIVER
REFLEX

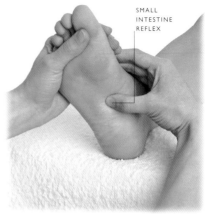

12 *Work the liver by caterpillar walking in a criss-cross manner. Hook up the gall bladder with the index finger.*

13 *Work the small-intestine by caterpillar walking in both horizontal directions.*

14 *Hook up the appendix and ileo-caecal reflex for a few seconds. Caterpillar walk up the ascending colon reflex and across the transverse colon reflex, ending at the instep of the right foot.*

ILEO-CAECAL
VALVE AND
APPENDIX REFLEX

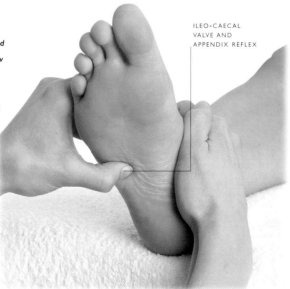

TIP
The reflexes for
the appendix and
the ileo-caecal valve
are at the same point
on the sole of the
right foot.

53

I5 *Work the bladder reflex by caterpillar walking diagonally up towards the little toe. The bladder, ureter, kidney and adrenal gland can be tender, so ask the client how they feel during this part of the treatment.*

TIP

A bladder reflex that is puffy and swollen in appearance indicates weakness in this important area of the body.

BLADDER REFLEX

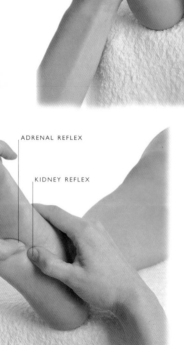

ADRENAL REFLEX

KIDNEY REFLEX

I6 *Work up the ureter reflex and the kidney reflex by caterpillar walking, stimulate the adrenal reflex, then work down the ureter reflex and the bladder reflex. Work the bladder reflex two or three times. The kidney and adrenal reflexes can both be stimulated together. This is done by placing one thumb on the kidney reflex and the other on the adrenal reflex, with the two thumbs facing each other. Pull the two thumbs away from one another, and then gently massage the reflexes with the thumbs for a few seconds.*

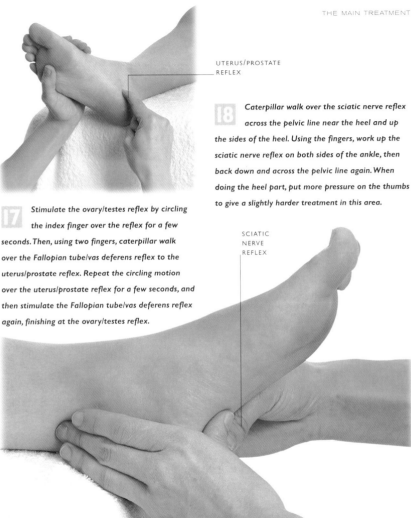

UTERUS/PROSTATE
REFLEX

18 Caterpillar walk over the sciatic nerve reflex across the pelvic line near the heel and up the sides of the heel. Using the fingers, work up the sciatic nerve reflex on both sides of the ankle, then back down and across the pelvic line again. When doing the heel part, put more pressure on the thumbs to give a slightly harder treatment in this area.

17 Stimulate the ovary/testes reflex by circling the index finger over the reflex for a few seconds. Then, using two fingers, caterpillar walk over the Fallopian tube/vas deferens reflex to the uterus/prostate reflex. Repeat the circling motion over the uterus/prostate reflex for a few seconds, and then stimulate the Fallopian tube/vas deferens reflex again, finishing at the ovary/testes reflex.

SCIATIC
NERVE
REFLEX

USE ALL FOUR
FINGERS

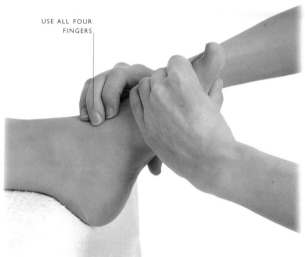

19 *Using all four
fingers, caterpillar
walk over the front of the
foot, starting at zone 5
and moving to zone 1.*

TIP
The breast
reflexes are located
on the front of both
feet. This part of the
treatment should be
very relaxing for
the client.

MASSAGE AROUND
ANKLE BONE

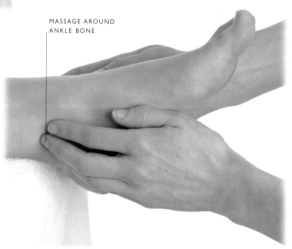

20 *Using your fingers,
gently massage around
the ankle bone – this is also a
reflex for the lymph of the
groin. Tenderness here relates to
pelvic inflammation.*

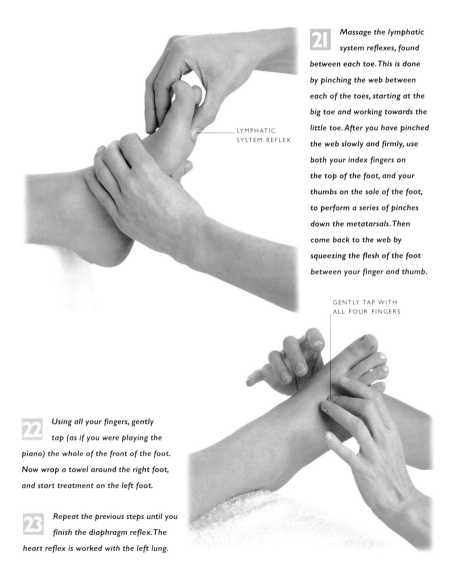

21 Massage the lymphatic system reflexes, found between each toe. This is done by pinching the web between each of the toes, starting at the big toe and working towards the little toe. After you have pinched the web slowly and firmly, use both your index fingers on the top of the foot, and your thumbs on the sole of the foot, to perform a series of pinches down the metatarsals. Then come back to the web by squeezing the flesh of the foot between your finger and thumb.

LYMPHATIC
SYSTEM REFLEX

GENTLY TAP WITH
ALL FOUR FINGERS

22 Using all your fingers, gently tap (as if you were playing the piano) the whole of the front of the foot. Now wrap a towel around the right foot, and start treatment on the left foot.

23 Repeat the previous steps until you finish the diaphragm reflex. The heart reflex is worked with the left lung.

SPLEEN
AND
STOMACH
REFLEX

SIGMOID
COLON
REFLEX

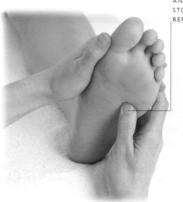

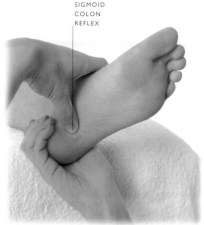

24 *Work the spleen and stomach reflex by caterpillar walking across zones 1 to 4.*

25 *Work the small intestine by caterpillar walking in both horizontal directions.*

26 *Caterpillar walk across the transverse colon reflex, down the descending colon reflex and along the sigmoid colon, dropping just below the pelvic line at the midline, then move up towards the bladder reflex. Squeeze the rectum reflex with your thumb.*

27 *Now work the rest of the left foot in a similar manner to the right foot.*

28 *When both feet have undergone the main treatment, the solar plexus relaxation treatment can be given. This relaxation method can also be given at the start of a treatment. The solar plexus is a network of nerves and the main storage area for stress. Applying pressure to this region always brings about a degree of relaxation.*

SMALL INTESTINE REFLEX

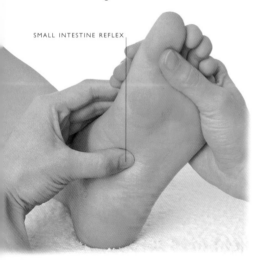

TIP
The solar plexus reflex can be seen on the foot as the apex of the arch running across the bottom of the ball of the foot.

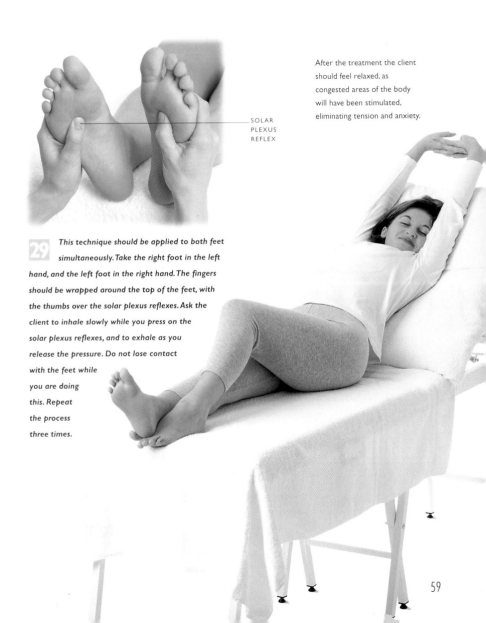

SOLAR
PLEXUS
REFLEX

After the treatment the client should feel relaxed, as congested areas of the body will have been stimulated, eliminating tension and anxiety.

29 *This technique should be applied to both feet simultaneously. Take the right foot in the left hand, and the left foot in the right hand. The fingers should be wrapped around the top of the feet, with the thumbs over the solar plexus reflexes. Ask the client to inhale slowly while you press on the solar plexus reflexes, and to exhale as you release the pressure. Do not lose contact with the feet while you are doing this. Repeat the process three times.*

59

Useful addresses

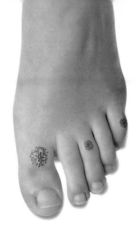

Association of Reflexologists
27 Old Gloucester Street
London
WC1N 3XX
Tel: 0870 5673320

Bayly School of Reflexology
Monks Orchard
Whitbourne
Worcs
WR6 5RB
Tel/Fax: 01886 821207
email: bayly@britreflex.co.uk
www.britreflex.co.uk

BCMA (British Complementary
Medicine Association)
33 Imperial Square
Cheltenham
Glos
GL0 1QZ
Tel: 0845 3455977
email: info@bcma.co.uk
www.bcma.co.uk

British School of Reflexology and Holistic
Association of Reflexologists
(BSR Sales Limited)
92 Sheering Road
Old Harlow
Essex
CM17 0JW
Tel: 01279 429066
Fax: 01279 445234
www.footreflexology.com

Chrysalis School of Reflexology
14 Central Avenue
Cookstown
County Tyrone
Northern Ireland
BT80 8AJ
Tel: 028 86763664

Colour and Reflexology
(contact: Pauline Wills)
9 Wyndale Avenue
Kingsbury
London
NW9 9PT
Tel/Fax: 020 82047672
email: pauline@oracleschoolstreet.co.uk

International Federation of Reflexologists
76–8 Edridge Road
Croydon
Surrey
CR0 1EF
Tel: 020 86679458
Fax: 020 86499291
www.reflexology-ifr.com

Irish Reflexologists' Institute
3 Blackglen Court
Lambs Cross
Sandyford
Dublin
Republic of Ireland

Scottish Institute of Reflexology
(contact: Margaret Whittington)
'Taymount'
Hill Crescent
Wormit
Fife
BD6 8PQ
Tel: 01382 541372

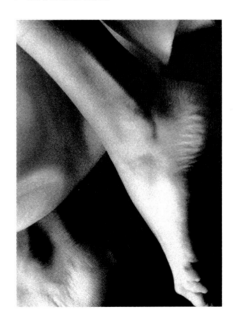

Glossary

ABDOMINAL AREA The area of the body that starts at the diaphragm and extends under the lungs to the genitals.

CARDIOVASCULAR Concerning the heart and/or the circulatory system.

CASE HISTORY This is where the therapist asks the client personal details, such as their medical history and occupation.

CONGESTION In reflexology this means an area of the body where there is not a free flow of energy.

HEALING CRISIS This is the process by which a patient gets rid of toxic substances, sometimes causing them to feel unwell.

HOLISTIC Taken from the Greek word *Holas*, which means 'whole'. In reflexology it means that the person is treated as a whole, on a physical, mental and spiritual level.

ORGAN A multicellular part of an animal, which forms a structural unit (e.g. the liver).

REFLEX An area found on the feet and hands that corresponds to a gland, an organ or a part of the body.

THORACIC AREA The area containing the heart and lungs. It is clearly marked off from the abdomen by the diaphragm.

TOXINS These are essentially poisons, which may be created by the body, ingested in the food we eat or drink or may enter the body by other means.

VITAL FORCE This is the same thing as the life force. It is the energy within us. Without it we cannot live.

WAISTLINE An imaginary line running horizontally across the foot and hand that relates to the real waistline (see pages 30–31).

ZONE In reflexology, any one of ten longitudinal sections through the body. Each zone contains one finger (or thumb) and one toe.

Finding a therapist

Reflexology has a number of regulatory boards. Any one of the organisations listed on pages 60–61 should be able to provide you with a list of registered practitioners. The following organisations also have members who are qualified reflexology practitioners.

International Institute of Reflexology UK
15 Hartfield Close
Tonbridge
Kent
TN10 4JP
Tel. 01732 350629

The Reflexogists Society
39 Prestbury Road
Cheltenham
Gloucester
GL52 2PT
Tel: 01242 512601

Many reflexologists work at health clinics. It is always worth checking their professional status and insurance cover.

Complaints

Always try to use a reflexologist who is a member of one of the regulatory boards. Then, should you have a complaint, the relevant board may be contacted.

Training Courses

If you wish to train as a therapist, any one of the organisations listed on pages 60–61 should be able to help.

The Association of Reflexologists is an independent organisation that is not affiliated to any particular training school, but it does publish a list of schools and training courses.